Atkins Diet for Women over 60

Easier Weight Loss with Atkins Diet Proven Strategies"

This book is designed to provide accurate and up-to-date information about the subject matter. It is sold with the understanding that the author and publisher are not providing medical, nutritional, or professional services. If you need expert assistance, please consult with a qualified healthcare or nutrition professional.

The author and publisher shall not be liable for any special, consequential, or exemplary damages resulting from the reader's use of, or reliance on, the information and recipes contained in this book.

By SOMTOOCHUKWU JUSTIN

About the Author

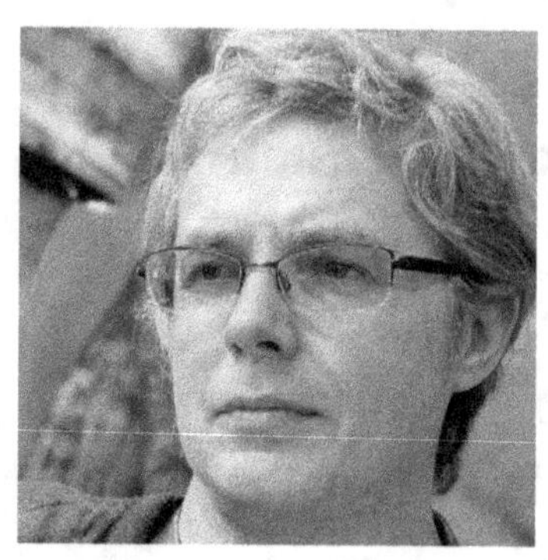

Somtoochukwu Justin is a recognized master in the field of well-being and health. With significant energy for working on the existence of Human health, he has committed his vocation to guarantee their well-being and satisfaction through sustenance and way-of-life decisions. Mr. Justin's broad information and experience make him a confided-in expert in the wellbeing and health area.

All through his vocation, Mr. Justin has worked indefatigably to elevate an all-encompassing way to deal with Health. He immovably accepts that smart dieting isn't just about sustaining the body yet in addition supporting the spirit. As the writer of "

Atkins diet for women over 60" he has nicely made a culinary aide that tends to the one-of-a-kind requirements of women, furnishing them with delicious, nutritious, and simple to-plan recipes.

Mr. Justin's obligation to women and men's well-being stretches out past his composition. He has been a devoted promoter of open and reasonable health sustenance, endeavoring to have a constructive outcome in the existence of men and women . His skill, sympathy, and immovable devotion to human wellbeing have made him a regarded figure in the wellbeing field, and his book is a demonstration of his obligation to working on the existence of health through the force of tasty and nutritious feasts some of his books includes _ **"afib healthy cookbook for men."** , **Easy Prepare Food For Seniors etc…**

Table of contents

Introduction:

Welcome to "Atkins Diet for Women over 60.This book is intended to be your confided in friend on the excursion to better wellbeing, customized to the extraordinary necessities of women in their sixties and then some. In the accompanying pages, I will investigate the Atkins Diet, a low-sugar way to deal with nourishment that has assisted endless people with accomplishing their weight, the executives and wellbeing objectives.

Customized Dietary Designs for women Over 60

As women age, their wholesome requirements change. The requests on their bodies and digestion systems develop, and what worked in the past may not be as viable any longer. This is where a customized dietary arrangement becomes fundamental.

women north of 60 frequently face explicit difficulties like hormonal variances, a diminished metabolic rate, and changing dietary inclinations. Subsequently, embracing a dietary methodology that considers these variables is significant.

My objective in this book is to furnish you with a dietary arrangement that thinks about the novel requirements and inclinations of women north of 60. We comprehend that one size doesn't fit all, and I mean to enable you to settle on decisions that are appropriate for your singular process.

Atkins Diet Principles

The Atkins Diet, which acquired fame many years prior, is grounded in the idea of carb limitation. It stresses decreasing your carb admission to move your body's essential energy source from carbs to put away fat.

The outcome? Weight reduction, further developed glucose control, and improved general prosperity.

In this book, I dig into the Atkins Diet standards, separating its different stages and making sense of how you can adjust and advance through them to accomplish your wellbeing and weigh the executives' objectives. We'll direct you through the excursion, beginning with the Acceptance Stage and advancing to the Upkeep Stage, assisting you with finding the right equilibrium of sugars that suits your body.

A Useful, Simple to-Follow, and Mentally Engaging Approach

The methodology is useful and simple to follow on the grounds that I comprehend that rolling out huge dietary improvements can feel overpowering. I've organized an assortment of flavorful and nutritious recipes explicitly intended for women more than 60, guaranteeing that each dish is both fulfilling and simple to plan. I've likewise given functional tips to dinner arranging and planning, so you can set out on this excursion with certainty.

Be that as it may, I go past the commonsense perspectives. This book is mentally engaging on the grounds that I realize that the weight of the executives and generally prosperity are not just about what you eat; they are likewise about how you think and feel. I'll investigate techniques to assist you with beating difficulties, remain propelled, and praise your triumphs. I'll dig into the brain science behind slimming down and proposition bits of knowledge on the most proficient method to keep a positive outlook.

The tone of this book is one of consolation and backing. I mean to enable you with the information and devices to assume command over your wellbeing and prosperity, regardless of your age. You are never too old to even consider leaving on an excursion to a better you.

Along these lines, how about we get everything rolling on this astonishing experience together. The way to better wellbeing, weight the board, and prosperity starts here, and I'm here to direct you constantly.

Part 1: Grasping the Atkins Diet

In this section, I will plunge into the essentials of the Atkins Diet, a dietary methodology that has endured over the extreme long haul and keeps on being an amazing asset for accomplishing weight for the executives and working on prosperity. I'll investigate the verifiable foundations of the eating regimen, its center standards, and the numerous ways fitting the particular requirements of women north of 60 can be adjusted.

The Atkins Diet is based on four unmistakable stages:

1. **Induction Phase:** This underlying stage limits carb admission to around 20-25 grams each day. During this stage, your body enters ketosis, and you'll encounter quick

weight reduction as it consumes fat for energy.

2. **Balancing Phase:** As you progress, you continuously once again introduce starches while checking your body's reaction. This stage assists you with recognizing your extraordinary degree of carb resistance, the place where you can keep on getting thinner while consuming somewhat more carbs.

3. **Pre-Upkeep and Support Phases:** In these stages, the center moves to keep up with your ideal weight. You keep on changing your carb consumption until you find the right equilibrium that keeps you in a solid weight territory without acquiring.

The Low-Carb Approach and Its Benefits

The center standard of the Atkins Diet is lessening carb consumption, especially refined sugars and starches. Thusly, you accomplish a few momentous advantages:

- **Weight Loss:** The low-carb approach is profoundly compelling for weight reduction. During ketosis, your body involves putting away fat for energy, bringing about an observable decrease in muscle to fat ratio.

- **Glucose Control:** Decreasing carbs can prompt more steady glucose levels, making the eating regimen engaging for people with diabetes or those in danger of fostering the condition.

- **Further developed Blood Lipid Profile:** Studies have shown that the Atkins Diet can prompt ideal changes in cholesterol levels, especially by expanding HDL (great) cholesterol and diminishing fatty oils.

- **Hunger Control:** Consuming protein and solid fats can assist you with feeling more full for longer, diminishing desires and the inclination to gorge.

Modifying the Atkins Diet for Individual Needs

What sets the Atkins Diet separated is its versatility. This diet perceives that every individual is one of a kind, and what works for one may not work for another. For women north of 60, customization is vital. Factors, for example, digestion, action level, and ailments can differ broadly, so the Atkins Diet can be custom-made to your particular requirements.

In the accompanying parts, I will direct you through the different periods of the Atkins Diet, telling you the best way to adjust and advance while considering your singular conditions. Whether your objective is weight reduction, better glucose control, or basically a better way of life, this diet can be a strong partner.

Understanding the standards and history of the Atkins Diet is the groundwork of your excursion. With this information, you'll be better prepared to pursue informed decisions and find how this low-carb approach can assist you with accomplishing your wellbeing and prosperity objectives as a lady north of 60.

Part 2: Exploring the Phases**

The Atkins Diet is certainly not a one-size-fits-all methodology, and it's pivotal to comprehend the different stages to successfully modify your excursion. In this part, I'll investigate the four essential periods of the Atkins Diet — Enlistment, Adjusting, Pre-Upkeep, and Support — diving into how women more than 60 can adjust to and progress through each stage and giving direction on setting customized carb limits.

1. Enlistment Phase

Purpose: The Enlistment Stage is the beginning stage, intended to launch your weight reduction by moving your body into ketosis. During this stage, starch admission is completely restricted to around 20-25 grams each day.

Transformation for women Over 60: It's vital to know that your metabolic rate might be slower than it was in your more youthful years. Thus, it could take somewhat longer to accomplish ketosis. Be encouraged by this. Remain committed, and you will see improvement. Guarantee that you stay very much hydrated and integrate low-influence practices that suit your wellness level.

Customized Carb Limit: During Enlistment, numerous women make progress with as far as possible. Notwithstanding, it's critical to pay attention to your body. Assuming that you find as far as possible excessively testing, think about expanding it somewhat yet guarantee you stay under 30 grams of net carbs each day.

2. Adjusting Phase

Purpose: The Adjusting Stage considers the continuous renewed introduction of starches to find your basic carb level for getting in shape. It's a customized stage to decide your ideal carb consumption.

Variation for women Over 60: More seasoned grown-ups may have a superior comprehension of their bodies and how they respond to different food sources. Utilize this for your potential benefit. Give close consideration to how your body answers as you once again introduce carbs. This stage is tied in with figuring out your perfect balance — where you keep on getting thinner yet can partake in a more shifted diet.

Customized Starch Limit: Start with a marginally higher carb consumption than during Enlistment, around 30-50 grams each day. Screen your headway intently and make changes depending on the situation. Try not to rush; find an opportunity to find what works for you.

3. Pre-Upkeep and Support Phases

Purpose: In these stages, the center moves to keep up with your ideal weight. You keep on changing your carb consumption until you find the right equilibrium that keeps you in a sound weight territory without acquiring.

Transformation for women Over 60: These stages are where your age and experience can genuinely sparkle. You might have a superior comprehension of what your body needs. Your objective here isn't just keeping a sound weight yet in addition supporting your general prosperity. Keep on being aware of carb consumption, yet remember to sustain your body with various supplements.

Customized Carb Limit: During Pre-Upkeep, you can expand your carb consumption bit by bit, going from 50-100 grams each day. For the Upkeep Stage, the breaking point may be associated with 100 grams or somewhat more. Pay attention to your body's signs and make changes depending on the situation to remain inside your objective weight territory.

Part3: Arranging and Preparation

Fruitful adherence to the Atkins Diet, particularly for women north of 60, frequently relies on successful preparation and readiness. In this part, I will investigate useful systems to assist you with exploring feast arranging, give an example week after week dinner plan, and stress the basic parts of piece control and following your starch consumption.

Functional Tips for Dinner Arranging and Preparation

1. **Create a Week after week Menu:** Start by arranging your feasts for the week. This recoveries you time and stress as well as guarantees that you have an assortment of delectable and low-carb choices.

2. **Grocery Shopping:** Set up a rundown in view of your menu. Adhere to your rundown to keep away from drive acquisition of high-carb things. Investigate the border of the store, which normally contains new produce, lean proteins, and dairy.

3. **Prep in Advance:** Invest energy on dinner prep throughout the end of the week or on a day that is helpful for you. Wash and cleave vegetables, cook proteins, and store them in segment estimated holders. This makes it simple to assemble a fast low-carb feast during the week.

4. **Stock Low-Carb Staples:** Keep your storage room and fridge loaded with Atkins-accommodating staples like olive oil, flavors, spices, nuts, seeds, and low-carb sauces. This guarantees you generally have the elements for a delicious, low-carb dinner.

5. **Mindful Eating:** Keep away from interruptions while eating, like sitting in front of the television or dealing with the PC. Find a seat at a table, bite your food gradually, and enjoy each nibble. This training can assist with segment control.

Test Week after week Feast Plan

Note: This is a fundamental example plan. You can adjust it in light of your inclinations and wholesome needs.

Day 1:
- **Breakfast:** Fried eggs with spinach and feta cheddar.
- **Lunch:** Barbecued chicken serving of mixed greens with blended greens and a vinaigrette dressing.
- **Snack:** Cucumber and cream cheddar chomps.

- **Dinner:** Prepared salmon with asparagus.

Day 2:
- **Breakfast:** Greek yogurt with berries and a sprinkle of nuts.
- **Lunch:** Turkey and avocado lettuce wraps.
- **Snack:** Celery sticks with peanut butter.
- **Dinner:** Meat pan sear with broccoli and cauliflower rice.

Day 3:
- **Breakfast:** Omelet with mushrooms, chime peppers, and cheddar.
- **Lunch:** Fish salad in lettuce cups.
- **Snack:** Almonds and string cheddar.
- **Dinner:** Cooked chicken with Brussels sprouts.

Day 4:

- **Breakfast:** Curds with cut peaches.
- **Lunch:** Spinach and bacon salad with a velvety farm dressing.
- **Snack:** Cut ringer peppers with guacamole.
- **Dinner:** Pork slashes with sautéed zucchini.

Day 5:
- **Breakfast:** Avocado and bacon breakfast sandwich.
- **Lunch:** Shrimp and avocado serving of mixed greens with a lemon spice dressing.
- **Snack:** Berries and whipped cream (sans sugar).
- **Dinner:** Barbecued steak with a side of green beans.

*Day 6 and 7:** Alter these days with your number one low-carb recipes and any eating out plans.

Segment Control and Following Starch Intake

- Use estimating cups and a food scale to guarantee you are eating proper piece sizes.
- Focus on food names to recognize the starch content in bundled food varieties.
- Consider keeping a food diary or utilizing a versatile application to follow your everyday carb consumption.
- As you progress through the stages, change your part measures and carb limits as per your customized plan.

Part 4: Delightful and Nutritious Recipes**

This section is devoted to giving a determination of mouth-watering low-carb recipes customized to the special wholesome requirements of women more than 60. These recipes are not difficult to plan and take care of various feasts over the course of the day, from breakfast to supper and, surprisingly, fulfilling snacks. I'll guarantee that each recipe adds to your prosperity and the support of a low-carb way of life, barring those irrelevant to your particular healthful necessities.

Breakfast Recipes

1. **Creamy Fried Eggs with Spinach and Feta:**

- A good breakfast that is rich in protein and sound fats, with an eruption of flavor from sautéed spinach and feta cheddar.

2. **Greek Yogurt Parfait with Berries and Nuts:**
   - A protein-stuffed and fulfilling breakfast that consolidates Greek yogurt with cell reinforcement rich berries and a sprinkle of heart-sound nuts.

3. **Avocado and Bacon Breakfast Sandwich:**
   - A great and filling low-carb breakfast with the velvety integrity of avocado and the exquisite mash of bacon.

Lunch Recipes

4. **Grilled Chicken Serving of mixed greens with Vinaigrette Dressing:**

- A light and reviving serving of mixed greens with barbecued chicken, blended greens, and a fiery vinaigrette dressing.

5. **Turkey and Avocado Lettuce Wraps:**
   - A basic and carb-cognizant lunch choice highlighting lean turkey and velvety avocado, enveloped by new lettuce leaves.

6. **Spinach and Bacon Salad with Smooth Farm Dressing:**
   - A tasty plate of mixed greens that joins the mash of bacon and the newness of spinach, finished off with a rich farm dressing.

Nibble Recipes

7. **Cucumber and Cream Cheddar Bites:**
   - A light and fulfilling nibble highlighting cucumber cuts and a spread of cream cheddar.

8. **Celery Sticks with Nut Butter:**
   - A crunchy and protein-pressed nibble joining the freshness of celery with the lavishness of peanut butter.

9. **Almonds and String Cheese:**
   - A compact bite that offers the energy of almonds and the richness of string cheddar.

Supper Recipes

10. **Baked Salmon with Asparagus:**
    - A nutritious and delightful supper with salmon as the star, supplemented by broiled asparagus.

11. **Beef Sautéed food with Broccoli and Cauliflower Rice:**
    - A low-carb curve on an exemplary sautéed food, highlighting delicate hamburger strips and fiber-rich vegetables.

12. **Roasted Chicken with Brussels Sprouts:**
   - A consoling supper with delicious cooked chicken and the natural kinds of Brussels sprouts.

These recipes are painstakingly chosen to meet your dietary necessities as a lady north of 60, advancing the two wellbeing and fulfillment. They underline the significance of flavor, assortment, and adjusted sustenance, guaranteeing that your low-carb venture is both delightful and nutritious.

Part 5: Mental Systems for Success

Outcome in taking on a dietary arrangement, especially for women north of 60, is as much a mental excursion as it is an actual one. In this section, I will dig into the brain science of slimming down and give you persuasive tips and methodologies to keep you on the way to progress. I'll investigate the meaning of positive self-talk and objective setting, and how these practices can be enabling and extraordinary.

Understanding the Brain research of Eating less junk food for women Over 60

Eating less junk food, regardless of the age, can be a perplexing and profound undertaking. women more than 60 frequently face one of a kind mental difficulties. It's urgent to recognize and address these perspectives to make your dietary process a positive and manageable one. A typical mental components to consider include:

1. **Self-Image:** As we age, self-perception can turn into a more huge element. Zeroing in on wellbeing and prosperity over esthetics is fundamental.

2. **Patience:** Weight reduction might happen at a slower speed for more seasoned grown-ups. Tolerance and sensible assumptions are indispensable.

3. **Social Dynamics:** Eating out and getting-togethers can sometimes present difficulties. Conveying your dietary necessities and limits can assist with exploring these circumstances.

4. **Emotional Eating:** Profound triggers for eating can be more perplexing as we age.

Figuring out how to perceive and deal with close to home eating is vital.

Inspirational Ways to remain on Track

1. **Set Sensible Goals:** Separate your drawn out objectives into more modest, feasible achievements. Commend every accomplishment to remain propelled.

2. **Find a Responsibility Partner:** Offering your excursion to a companion or relative can offer truly necessary help and inspiration.

3. **Mindful Eating:** Focus on your body's yearning and completion signs. Eating carefully can assist you with trying not to indulge and pursue better decisions.

4. **Positive Reinforcement:** Utilize positive insistences and prize yourself

(without nourishment) for arriving at achievements. Indulge yourself with something you appreciate, similar to a spa day or another book.

The Force of Positive Self-Talk and Objective Setting

1. **Positive Self-Talk:** The words you use to depict your process are strong. Rather than saying, "I can't," say, "I decide not to." Shift your mentality from humility to self-strengthening. Practice self-empathy and help yourself to remember your advancement.

2. **Goal-Setting:** Setting clear, attainable objectives can keep you engaged and inspired. These objectives ought to be explicit, quantifiable, and time-bound. For example, rather than saying, "I need to get in

shape," say, "I mean to shed 10 pounds in the following three months."

3. **Visualize Your Success:** Picturing your prosperity can be an intense inspiration. Make a psychological picture of your better, more joyful self and utilize this picture as a wellspring of motivation.

4. **Keep a Journal:** Think about keeping a diary to record your contemplations, sentiments, and progress. Journaling can give important bits of knowledge into your excursion.

5. **Stay Flexible:** Recall that mishaps are a characteristic piece of any excursion. It's alright to have off days, yet the key is to continue to push ahead.

By understanding the mental elements of eating fewer carbs for women north of 60 and embracing the force of positive self-talk and objective setting, you can upgrade your excursion towards better wellbeing and prosperity.

Part 6: Beating Challenges**

Setting out on the Atkins Diet as a lady north of 60 can be a compensating venture, yet like any undertaking, it's not without its difficulties. In this part, I will address the normal obstacles looked by women in this age group on the Atkins Diet and give procedures to assist you with exploring these difficulties effectively. I will examine how to deal with social circumstances, oversee desires, and defeat levels, all while stressing the significance of self-sympathy and versatility.

Normal Difficulties Looked by women More than 60 on the Atkins Diet

1. **Slower Metabolism:** As you age, your digestion might dial back, making weight reduction really testing. This can be disappointing, however recall that progress is

as yet conceivable, though at an alternate speed.

2. **Social Situations:** Eating out with loved ones or going to get-togethers can be precarious while sticking to a particular dietary arrangement. Imparting your dietary requirements and looking for steady environments is fundamental.

3. **Cravings:** Desires for high-carb food varieties can be particularly relentless for women north of 60. Dealing with these desires and finding fulfilling low-carb options can be a huge test.

4. **Plateaus:** Weight reduction levels can happen on any eating regimen. It tends to be dispiriting when the scale doesn't move, however levels are a typical piece of the weight reduction process. They are normally

transitory and can frequently be overwhelmed with perseverance.

Techniques for Dealing with Challenges

1. **Slower Metabolism:** Be patient and embrace the excursion. Comprehend that more slow weight reduction doesn't compare to an absence of progress. Center around non-scale triumphs like expanded energy, further developed glucose control, and upgraded prosperity.

2. **Social Situations:** Impart your dietary necessities to people around you. The vast majority are steady once they figure out your objectives. In the event that you're going to a get-together, propose to bring a low-carb dish to share.

3. **Cravings:** Recognize your trigger food sources and supplant them with

low-carb choices. Hankering something sweet? Decide on berries with whipped cream. Hankering crunchy? Appreciate cucumber cuts with plunge. Recall that desires frequently pass assuming you occupy yourself with a drawing in movement or basically stand by a couple of moments.

4. **Plateaus:** When you hit a weight reduction level, consider rethinking your carb admission and work-out daily practice. Here and there, gaining minor changes can reignite your headway. In particular, recall that levels are transitory, and timelessness pays off.

Self-Empathy and Resilience

At long last, rehearsing self-sympathy and versatility all through your journey is pivotal. Recognize that mishaps and difficulties are an ordinary piece of any undertaking. Be thoughtful to yourself when you face snags, and on second thought of harping on apparent disappointments, center around your triumphs and progress.

Flexibility is your capacity to adjust and return quickly from difficulties. As a lady more than 60, you've previously exhibited versatility all through your life. Apply that solidarity to your dietary process. Recollect that you have the inward assets to beat difficulties and remain focused.

Part 7: Remaining Dynamic and Healthy

A far reaching way to deal with wellbeing and prosperity includes something other than dietary decisions. Standard actual work is a basic part, particularly for women north of 60. In this part, I will investigate the significance of activity, recommend age-proper wellness schedules, and talk about the advantages of consolidating the Atkins Diet with actual work to upgrade your general wellbeing and health.

The Significance of Ordinary Activity for women Over 60

Practice is a vital component of keeping a sound way of life as you age. It offers a great many advantages, including:

1. **Weight Management:** Ordinary activity assists with consuming calories and constructing muscle, making it a fundamental apparatus for weight the executives and forestalling weight gain.

2. **Bone Health:** Weight-bearing activities, for example, strolling and opposition preparing, advance bone thickness and can lessen the gamble of osteoporosis.

3. **Cardiovascular Health:** Actual work helps bring down the gamble of coronary illness, stroke, and hypertension by working on cardiovascular wellbeing.

4. **Mood and Mental Health:** Exercise discharges endorphins, which can upgrade your state of mind, lessen pressure, and work on mental prosperity.

5. **Flexibility and Balance:** Keeping up with adaptability and equilibrium through exercises like yoga and extending can forestall wounds and falls.

Age-Fitting Wellness Routines

Exercise ought to be custom-made to your singular wellness level, interests, and state of being. As a lady north of 60, consider these age-suitable wellness schedules:

1. **Aerobic Activities:** Low-influence exercises like strolling, swimming, and cycling are fantastic for cardiovascular wellbeing without overburdening joints.

2. **Strength Training:** Incorporate strength preparing practices utilizing light loads, opposition groups, or body weight to assemble and keep up with bulk.

3. **Yoga and Pilates:** These practices upgrade adaptability, equilibrium, and center strength, making them helpful for generally speaking prosperity.

4. **Tai Chi:** A sluggish, thoughtful practice that further develops equilibrium, adaptability, and mental concentration.

5. **Functional Fitness:** Activities that emulate everyday exercises, like squats, jumps, and step-ups, can work on useful strength.

Joining the Atkins Diet with Actual Activity

The collaboration between the Atkins Diet and actual work is strong. Practice supplements the eating regimen in more ways than one:

1. **Enhanced Weight Loss:** Joining a low-carb diet with ordinary activity can prompt more huge weight reduction than consuming less calories alone.

2. **Improved Metabolism:** Exercise can support digestion, assisting your body with consuming calories all the more proficiently.

3. **Blood Sugar Control:** Active work can further develop insulin awareness and help in better glucose control.

4. **Stress Reduction:** Exercise is a powerful pressure reliever, which is particularly significant for women north of 60 who might be managing pressure related medical problems.

5. **Better Mental Health:** The mind-set upgrading advantages of activity can add to a

positive outlook, which is significant for adherence to the eating routine.

Recall that it's critical to talk with a medical care supplier prior to starting another activity program, particularly assuming you have any basic ailments. Your medical services supplier can give direction and proposals in view of your singular wellbeing and wellness needs.

Part 8: Remaining Hydrated and Overseeing Supplements**

In this part, I will investigate the significance of remaining sufficiently hydrated and overseeing supplements as a lady more than 60 on the Atkins Diet. Legitimate hydration, alongside proper supplementation, assumes a crucial part in supporting your weight, the executives and in general wellbeing.

The Meaning of Hydration in Weight Management

Hydration is in many cases misjudged in its part in the weight of the board. Here's the reason it's fundamental:

1. **Appetite Control:** Now and again, thirst can be confused with hunger. Remaining very much hydrated can assist

you with separating between the two and forestall superfluous nibbling.

2. **Metabolism Support:** Sufficient water admission is fundamental for keeping a solid digestion. Indeed, even gentle drying out can dial back metabolic cycles.

3. **Digestive Health:** Water is essential for the processing and assimilation of supplements. Appropriate assimilation supports the weight of the executives.

4. **Exercise Performance:** Remaining hydrated is critical to compelling exercises. Legitimate hydration upholds muscle capability and perseverance during exercise.

5. **Detoxification:** Water assists your body with taking out waste and poisons, further advancing prosperity.

Suggested Enhancements for More established Women

Enhancements can assist with filling healthful holes, particularly as we age. Here are a few suggested supplements for more seasoned ladies:

1. **Multivitamins:** A great multivitamin can guarantee you get fundamental nutrients and minerals. Search for one intended for women north of 60.

2. **Vitamin D:** Numerous more established grown-ups have lower levels of vitamin D, which is crucial for bone wellbeing. Your medical services supplier can assist with deciding the right measurement.

3. **Calcium:** To keep up major areas of strength for and lessen the gamble of osteoporosis.

4. **Omega-3 Greasy Acids:** These can uphold heart wellbeing and decrease aggravation.

5. **Probiotics:** These are advantageous for stomach related wellbeing, which can some of the time become more touchy with age.

6. **B12:** As we age, the body's capacity to retain vitamin B12 from food reduces. Enhancements can assist with forestalling lack.

Pragmatic Ways to keep up with Generally Health

1. **Set a Hydration Goal:** Hold back nothing 8-10 cups of water a day, and change in view of your movement level and environment.

2. **Balance Electrolytes:** While following a low-carb diet, it's vital to keep up with the equilibrium of electrolytes like sodium, potassium, and magnesium. Talk with your medical care supplier about supplementation, if necessary.

3. **Consult with a Medical care Provider:** Prior to beginning any new enhancements or rolling out critical dietary improvements, talk with a medical care supplier. They can give customized proposals in view of your wellbeing needs and objectives.

4. **Whole Food varieties First:** Whenever the situation allows, get your fundamental supplements from entire food sources as

opposed to supplements. A reasonable eating routine is the groundwork of good wellbeing.

5. **Listen to Your Body:** Focus on indications of lack of hydration, like dull pee or dry mouth. These are signals that you really want more liquids.

Part 9: Looking for Help and Building a Community

Leaving on a dietary excursion, for example, the Atkins Diet, can be a groundbreaking encounter, yet it doesn't need to be a lone one. In this section, I will investigate the huge worth of encouraging groups of people and responsibility accomplices for women north of 60. I will recommend ways of interfacing with similar people and urge women to impart their excursion and encounters to others in a comparable way.

The Worth of Encouraging groups of people and Responsibility Partners

Encouraging groups of people and responsibility accomplices assume an essential part in accomplishing and keeping up with your wellbeing and prosperity objectives. Here's the reason they are fundamental:

1. **Motivation:** Backing from others can be a strong inspiration. It's reassuring to impart your excursion to the people who figure out your difficulties and wins.

2. **Accountability:** Knowing that you're responsible to another person can assist you with remaining focused on your dietary and wellness objectives.

3. **Inspiration:** Catching wind of the examples of overcoming adversity and encounters of others can be exceptionally moving, giving a feeling of local area and mutual perspective.

4. **Emotional Support:** Counting calories and way of life changes can be a sincere challenge. Having an encouraging group of

people gives a place of refuge to discuss your thoughts and get support.

Ways Of associating with Similar Individuals

1. **Online Communities:** There are various internet based networks and discussions where you can associate with people who are additionally on their wellbeing and health venture. Virtual entertainment stages and devoted sites offer spaces for conversation and backing.

2. **Local Backing Groups:** Search for nearby care groups or meet-ups in your space. Numerous people groups have bunches that emphasize on wellbeing and health, including those revolving around low-carb slims down like Atkins.

3. **Fitness Classes:** Joining wellness classes or gatherings custom fitted to your inclinations can assist you with interfacing with similar people who are likewise dedicated to a solid way of life.

4. **Reaching Out to Companions and Family:** In some cases, those nearest to you can turn into your best encouraging group of people. Share your objectives and progress with loved ones, and inquire as to whether they might want to go along with you in your excursion.

Empowering women to Share Their Excursion and Experiences

Sharing your excursion and encounters can be compensating for yourself as well as for others too. Here's the reason it's significant:

1. **Empowerment:** By sharing your story, you engage yourself and move others to assume command over their wellbeing and prosperity.

2. **Accountability:** Imparting your objectives and progress to others makes a feeling of responsibility. You're bound to adhere to your arrangement when others know about it.

3. **Problem Solving:** Discussing your difficulties can prompt arrangements. Others might offer experiences or systems they've tracked down viable in comparative circumstances.

4. **Community:** Building a feeling of local area and common help can be improving and satisfying.

Your encounters, experiences, and victories are interesting and important. By sharing them, you add to a developing local area of people committed to a better way of life. You rouse and engage people around you to assume responsibility for their prosperity, making a far reaching influence of inspiration and change.

Part 10: Observing Success**

Praising your prosperity is an imperative piece of your excursion on the Atkins Diet. It's a method for recognizing your accomplishments, both of all shapes and sizes, and keeping up with your inspiration as long as possible. In this part, I will give thoughts to non-food compensations to celebrate achievements, share examples of overcoming adversity of women more than 60 who have blossomed with the Atkins Diet, and build up the possibility that age isn't a hindrance to accomplishing wellbeing and weight objectives.

Thoughts for Non-Food Rewards

Rather than involving food as a prize for your achievements, consider these non-food ways of commending your triumphs:

1. **Spa Day:** Indulge yourself with a loosening up back rub, facial, or spa day. It's an extraordinary way to de-stress and spoil yourself.

2. **New Wardrobe:** When you arrive at a huge achievement, purchase another dress thing that you love and that accommodates your evolving body.

3. **Fitness Gear:** Put resources into some great exercise gear, for example, agreeable shoes, exercise garments, or hardware like obstruction groups or a wellness tracker.

4. **Personalized Jewelry:** Consider getting a piece of gems engraved with a significant message or the date of your prosperity.

5. **Adventure or Experience:** Plan an undertaking like a sight-seeing balloon ride, a climbing trip, or a visit to another objective.

6. **Learning Opportunity:** Sign up for a class or studio to discover some new information or foster an expertise you've without exception needed to dominate.

7. **Book or Individual Development:** Buy a book that rouses you or consider a self-improvement course.

Examples of overcoming adversity of women Over 60

The following are a couple of helpful examples of overcoming adversity from women more than 60 who have blossomed with the Atkins Diet:

1. Susan's Rousing Process at 62:

At 62, Susan had battled with her weight for the vast majority of her life. She chose to check the Atkins Diet out in the wake of finding out about its viability. Susan's obligation to a low-carb way of life drove her to shed 50 pounds throughout the span of a year. She shed pounds as well as saw huge enhancements in her circulatory strain and cholesterol levels. Today, Susan partakes in a functioning and satisfying retirement, voyaging and investigating new leisure activities she once believed were far off.

2. Tune's Change at 68:

After her retirement at 68, Ditty concluded the time had come to zero in on her wellbeing. She embraced the Atkins Diet and left on an excursion that saw her shed 40 pounds. All the more significantly, she acquired a freshly discovered feeling of imperativeness and self-assurance. Song's moving story fills in as a demonstration of the way that age is no snag to accomplishing critical wellbeing and health objectives.

3. Margaret's Dynamic Way of life at 63:

Margaret, at 63, had confronted difficulties with versatility and energy. In the wake of taking on the Atkins Diet, she encountered a momentous change. She shed 35 pounds and felt more lively than she had in years. This freshly discovered essentialness urged Margaret to investigate new leisure activities, and she currently appreciates cultivating, climbing, and, surprisingly, taking dance classes. Her story shows that earnestly and the right dietary arrangement, embracing an energetic and dynamic lifestyle is rarely past the point of no return.

4. Patricia's Excursion at 65:

Patricia, at 65, chose to assume command over her well being after a diabetes conclusion. She started following the Atkins Diet under the direction of her medical care supplier. Over the long haul, Patricia shed 30 pounds and, above all, accomplished better control of her glucose. Her excursion worked on her actual wellbeing as well as supported her certainty and personal satisfaction.

5. Betty's Wellbeing Change at 66:

Betty, at 66, had battled with joint torment and portability issues. She went to the Atkins Diet for an answer. Throughout a year, Betty shed 45 pounds, which fundamentally mitigated the stress on her joints. She additionally found herself ready to appreciate exercises like climbing and moving, which she hadn't done in years. Betty's story outlines the force of a low-carb way of life in working on weight as well as generally health.

6. Anne's Essentialness Revived at 70:

Anne, at, not entirely settled to improve with age and steadily. She took on the Atkins Diet and shed 25 pounds, however what was much more momentous was the flood of energy and mental lucidity she acquired. Anne wound up seeking after her energy for painting and chipping in for nearby causes, encapsulating the idea that age is no hindrance to a functioning and satisfying life.

7. Sarah's Excursion to Reestablished Certainty at 63:

At 63, Sarah concluded the time had come to recover her certainty and work on her wellbeing. She set out on the Atkins Diet and shed 40 pounds throughout a year. Past the weight reduction, Sarah discovered another healthy identity affirmation. She began chasing after exercises she had procrastinated on for a really long time and, most outstandingly, joined a neighborhood theater bunch. Her story embodies how a low-carb way of life can change your body as well as your confidence and self-awareness.

8. Emily's Weight reduction and Further developed Glucose at 61:

Emily, at 61, had long struggled with her weight and high glucose. She went to the Atkins Diet for help and shed 35 pounds. Her wonderful achievement likewise converted into better glucose control, which was a unique advantage for her wellbeing. Emily's story represents what dietary decisions can have a significant meaning for overseeing persistent medical issues.

9. Linda's Dynamic Retirement at 68:

Linda, at 68, resigned with dreams of a functioning and satisfying retirement. She focused on the Atkins Diet and, over the long haul, shed 45 pounds. This weight reduction permitted her to have a functioning existence loaded up with movement, climbing, and investing quality energy with her grandkids. Linda's process advises us that age is a chance to embrace life's experiences with excitement.

10. Jane's Weight reduction and Lively Retirement at 69:

Jane, at, not entirely settled to lead a lively and dynamic retirement. She embraced the Atkins Diet and, north of a year, shed 50 pounds. The weight reduction worked on her wellbeing as well as her portability. Jane currently appreciates everyday strolls, moving, and voyaging, demonstrating that age is no obstruction to a satisfying and dynamic way of life.

11. Martha's Victory Over Wellbeing Difficulties at 64:

Martha, at 64, confronted different wellbeing challenges, including hypertension and joint torment. She took on the Atkins Diet for the purpose of working on her wellbeing. In the span of a year, Martha shed 35 pounds, essentially diminishing the stress on her joints and really dealing with her circulatory strain. Her process shows the way that rolling out dietary improvements can significantly affect generally speaking prosperity.

12. Ruth's Reestablished Energy and Wellness at 67:

At 67, Ruth was looking for a reestablished feeling of energy and wellness. She focused on the Atkins Diet and over the long run shed 40 pounds. All the more significantly, her energy levels took off, permitting her to investigate new proactive tasks, including yoga and swimming. Ruth's story underlines that age ought as far as possible your quest for a functioning and empowering life.

These accounts delineate the inconceivable capability of the Atkins Diet for ladies north of 60. They grandstand the limit with regards to positive change, whether it's recovering essentialness in retirement, winning over wellbeing challenges, or appreciating recently discovered wellness. These ladies' encounters act as a wake up call that it's never beyond any good time to leave on an excursion towards better wellbeing and prosperity through the Atkins Diet.

Age Isn't a Boundary to Accomplishing Wellbeing and Weight Goals

Age ought to never be viewed as a hindrance to accomplishing your wellbeing and weight objectives. Your body has an unimaginable limit with respect to change, paying little heed to how long you've lived. The Atkins Diet is versatile and viable for women north of 60, and the examples of overcoming adversity of others in your age group are confirmation of that.

Praise each step of your excursion, regardless of how little, and keep laying out new objectives for yourself. Recollecting that achievement isn't just about arriving at a particular number on the scale; it's tied in with further developing your general prosperity, partaking in your life, and feeling certain and great.

Age isn't a hindrance; it's a potential chance to flourish.

Conclusion

As we draw the last section of this book to a close, it's fundamental to consider the groundbreaking excursion you've left on as a lady north of 60 looking for a better, low-carb way of life through the Atkins Diet. Here are the vital focal points and a last expression of motivation and support.

Key Takeaways

1. **Personalized Approach:** The Atkins Diet is definitely not a one-size-fits-all arrangement. It's tied in with tweaking the eating regimen to your extraordinary necessities and inclinations, guaranteeing a reasonable and pleasant way to wellbeing and prosperity.

2. **Mindset Matters:** The mental parts of your process are just about as fundamental as the actual ones. Developing a positive outlook, rehearsing self-sympathy, and defining sensible objectives are all keys to progress.

3. **Support and Community:** Building an encouraging group of people, finding responsibility accomplices, and imparting your excursion to others can enormously upgrade your inspiration and results.

4. **Healthy Aging:** Age isn't an obstruction to accomplishing your wellbeing and weight objectives. The motivating accounts of women north of 60 blossoming with the Atkins Diet show that change is conceivable at whatever stage in life.

5. **Holistic Wellness:** Accomplishing wellbeing and prosperity isn't exclusively

about weight reduction. About embracing an all encompassing methodology incorporates hydration, exercise, enhancements, and taking care of oneself.

A Last Expression of Inspiration

Embracing a better, low-carb way of life as a lady north of 60 isn't just about the objective; it's about the actual excursion. Your way to prosperity is a demonstration of your inward strength, versatility, and obligation to taking care of oneself. Recollect that age isn't an impediment; it's a potential chance to flourish, develop, and keep composing the narrative of your existence with wellbeing, essentialness, and satisfaction.

As you push ahead, convey with you the information that you have the apparatuses and the help to succeed. Praise every achievement, both of all shapes and sizes, and consistently remember your drawn out prosperity. The Atkins Diet is definitely not a handy solution; it's an economical, versatile, and satisfying way of life.

 it's not just about the weight you lose; it's about the existence you gain. Embrace the excursion, commend your triumphs, and keep on focusing on your prosperity. You have the ability to carry on with a day to day existence that is sound, energetic, and loaded up with potential outcomes.

Appendices**

In this segment, you'll find important assets, extra low-carb recipes, and feast arranging apparatuses to help your excursion. There's likewise a space for individual notes and reflections, permitting you to tailor your experience and keep tabs on your development.

1. Assets for Additional Data and Support

- **Websites:** Investigate legitimate sites committed to the Atkins Diet and low-carb residing, where you can track down articles, recipes, and gatherings for local area support.

- **Books:** Search for books by specialists in the field of low-carb living and sound maturing for additional experiences and direction.

- **Medical care Providers:** Your medical services supplier can offer customized guidance, backing, and proposals for your one of a kind wellbeing needs.

- **Social Media:** Join important virtual entertainment gatherings and follow accounts committed to low-carb living and wellbeing and health. These people can offer important experiences and inspiration.

- **Nearby Help Groups:** If accessible in your space, consider joining neighborhood wellbeing and health support gatherings to associate with similar people.

2. Extra Low-Carb Recipes and Feast Arranging Tools

- Find an assortment of extraordinary failure carb recipes to keep your dinners fascinating and delightful. Explore different avenues regarding various fixings and flavors to find what suits your preferences and dietary objectives.

- Access feast arranging instruments, for example, shopping records and dinner schedules, to assist you with remaining coordinated and on target with your dietary arrangement.

3. Individual Notes and Reflections

Utilize this space to record your own contemplations, progress, and reflections on your excursion. Report your achievements, challenges you've survived, and the examples you've advanced en route. These notes can be a wellspring of inspiration and knowledge as you keep on embracing a better, low-carb way of life.

Recollect that your process is extraordinary, and these indices are intended to improve your experience and furnish you with the devices and data you want to prevail on the Atkins Diet and your way to better wellbeing and prosperity.

APPRECIATION

**Thank you for reaching the end of this
journey with me, I know you enjoy it.**

**I'm looking forward to seeing your nice
and encouraging reviews!!**

**<u>Check out for more of my interesting
books!</u>**